TOP 50 YOGA POSES

Carl Preston

© 2015 Carl Preston

Edited by: Carl Preston

Cover by: Carl Preston

All rights reserved. No part of this publication may be reproduced, stored in a retrieval system, or transmitted in any form or by any means, electronic, mechanical, recording or otherwise, without the prior written permission of the author.

Whydontyouchange.com   2015

First Edition

DISCLAIMER

This book details the author's personal experiences with and opinions about right-brained learning. The author is not licensed as an educational consultant, teacher, psychologist, or psychiatrist.

The author and publisher are providing this book and its contents on an "as is" basis and make no representations or warranties of any kind with respect to this book or its contents. The author and publisher disclaim all such representations and warranties, including for example warranties of merchantability and educational or medical advice for a particular purpose. In addition, the author and publisher do not represent or warrant that the information accessible via this book is accurate, complete or current.

The statements made about products and services have not been evaluated by the U.S. government. Please consult with your own legal or accounting professional regarding the suggestions and recommendations made in this book.

Except as specifically stated in this book, neither the author or publisher, nor any authors, contributors, or other representatives will be liable for damages arising out of or in connection with the use of this book. This is a comprehensive limitation of liability that applies to all damages of any kind, including (without limitation) compensatory; direct, indirect or consequential damages; loss of data, income or profit; loss of or damage to property and claims of third parties.

You understand that this book is not intended as a substitute for consultation with a licensed medical, educational, legal or accounting professional. Before you begin any change in your lifestyle in any way, you will consult a licensed professional to ensure that you are doing what's best for your situation.

This book provides content related to educational, medical, and psychological topics. As such, use of this book implies your acceptance of this disclaimer.

Table of Contents

1 TOP 50 YOGA POSES 7

THE TIGER POSE 7

THE STANDING KNEE TO CHEST BALANCE 8

THE GAS RELEASE POSE 9

THE BOAT POSE 10

THE CORPSE POSE 11

THE THUNDERBOLT POSE 12

THE NOBLE POSE 13

THE SEATED FORWARD FOLD POSE 14

THE BOUND ANGLE POSE 15

THE MOUNTAIN POSE 16

THE PLOW POSE 17

THE TRIANGLE POSE 18

THE HEAD STAND POSE 19

THE SHOULDER STAND POSE 20

THE LOWER BACK TWIST 21

THE EASY BRIDGE POSE 22

THE CROCODILE POSE 23

THE STANDING KNEE SIDE BALANCE POSE 24

THE CHAIR POSE 25

THE REVOLVED SIDE ANGLE STRETCH POSE 26

THE ONE LEG FORWARD BEND POSE I 27

THE ONE LEG FORWARD BEND POSE II 28

THE WARRIOR POSE I 29

THE WARRIOR POSE II 30

THE WARRIOR POSE III 31

THE LOTUS POSE 32

THE BOUND ANGLE POSE 33
THE FISH POSE 34
THE BUTTERFLY POSE 35
THE TWISTED FORWARD STRETCH POSE 36
THE LOCUST POSE 37
THE BOW POSE 38
THE COBRA POSE 39
THE CHILD POSE 40
THE CAT POSE 41
THE DOWNWARD FACING DOG POSE 42
THE RAISED LEG DOWNWARD FACING DOG POSE 43
THE TIPTOE POSE 44
THE CHEST EXPAND POSE 45
THE SIDE PLANK POSE 46
THE DOLPHIN POSE 47
THE SURRENDER POSE 48
THE EXTENDED SIDE ANGLE STRETCH POSE 49
THE WIDE LEG FORWARD BEND POSE 50
THE HALF MOON POSE 51
THE RABBIT POSE 52
THE HEAD TO KNEE POSE WITH STRETCHING POSE 53
THE STANDING BOW PULLING POSE 54
THE HALF TORTOISE POSE 55
THE BALANCING STICK POSE 56

2   WEEK SCHEDULE TO INCREASE RELAXATION 57
3   WEEK SCHEDULE TO INCREASE FLEXIBILITY 58
4   WEEK SCHEDULE TO IMPROVE BREATHING 60
5   WEEK SCHEDULE TO INCREASE MENTAL FOCUS 61

1 TOP 50 YOGA POSES

THE TIGER POSE

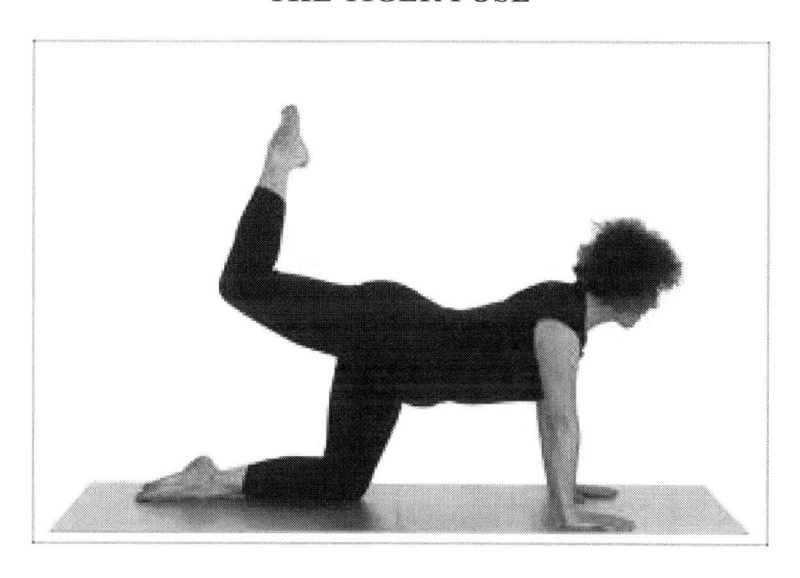

The tiger pose helps to relieve pains affecting the back, hip and outer side of the leg and loosens up the hip and legs joints. It also exercises and loosens the back by bending it alternately in both directions, harmonizing the spinal nerves. It stretches the abdominal muscles hence promoting digestion and stimulating blood circulation. It could also reduce weight from the hips and thighs

THE STANDING KNEE TO CHEST BALANCE

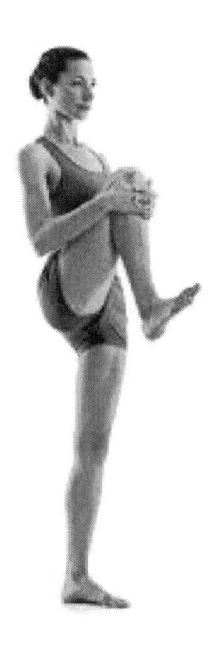

The Standing knee to chest balance helps to keep the abdominal muscles and nerves toned. It stretches the abdominal muscles and the intestines, hence helps in stimulating digestion. It also helps to build up mental and physical balance. The pose also improves the posture and strengthening the muscles in the arms.

THE GAS RELEASE POSE

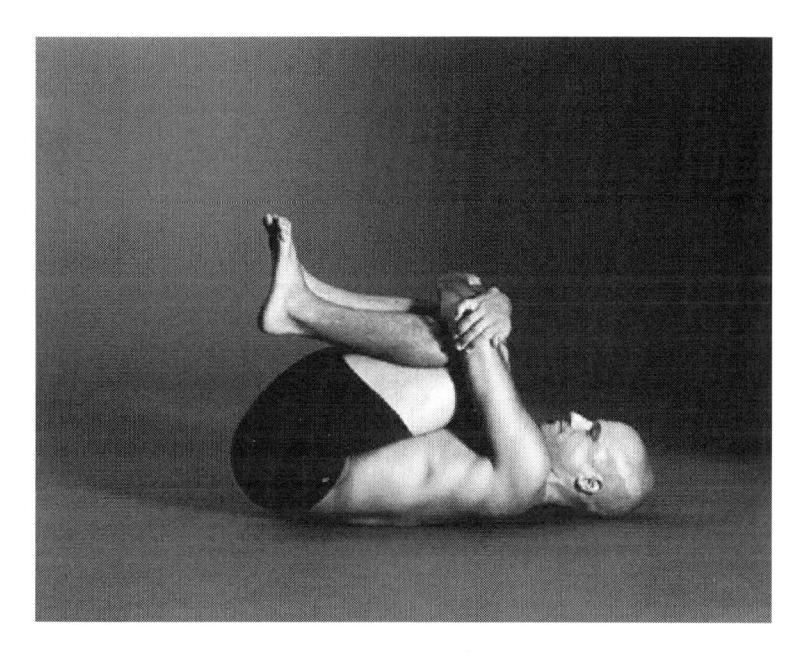

The gas release pose is just the thing pose for getting rid of wind and constipation since it massages the abdomen and the digestive organs. It loosens the spinal vertebrae and also strengthens the neck and lower back. It also assists in improving digestion and hence increases blood circulation in abdominal organs.

THE BOAT POSE

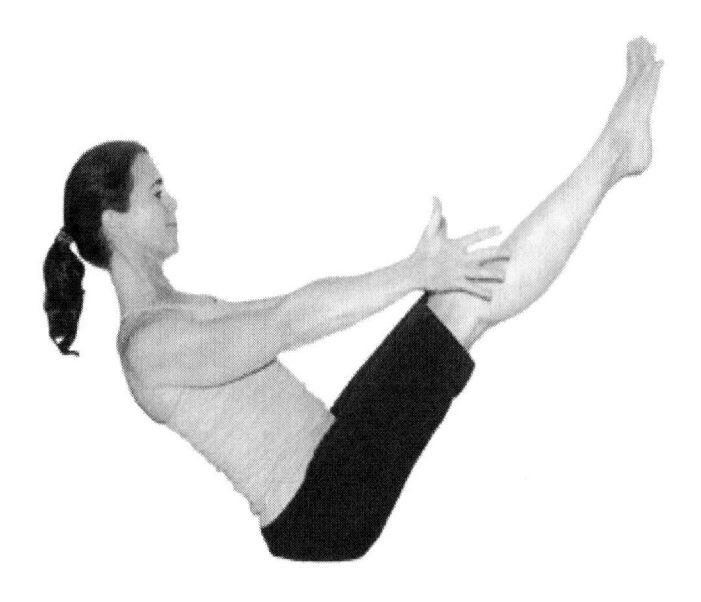

This pose is particularly useful for getting rid of nervous tension and bringing about deep relaxation. It stimulates the muscular, digestive, circulatory, nervous and hormonal systems, tones all the organs and removes weariness. It strengthens the intestine, removes constipation, gas formation, and obesity. It helps to relieve stomach pain. It is also useful for persons suffering from weak nerves and tension.

THE CORPSE POSE

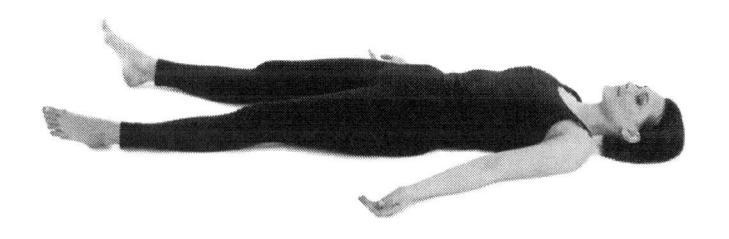

The corpse pose is very helpful for calming down the mind which is important for meditation. It lightens up the body and enhances responsiveness of the mind. It reduces high blood pressure. It helps in recovering from summer heat exhaustion and hypertension. This will help in controlling large number of diseases caused by tension.

THE THUNDERBOLT POSE

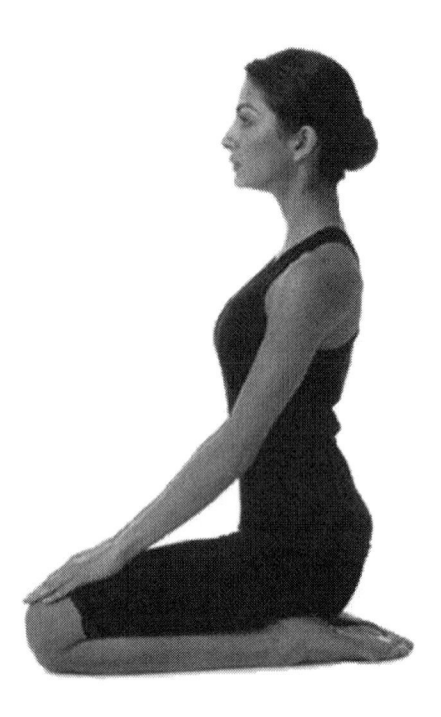

The pose is the best meditation pose for people suffering from sacral infections. It relieves stomach ailment such as hyperacidity and peptic ulcer and strengthens the pelvic muscles which is a preventative measure against hernia and helps to relieve piles. It helps in the treatment of dilated testicles in men and assists women in labor and helps ease menstrual disorders.

THE NOBLE POSE

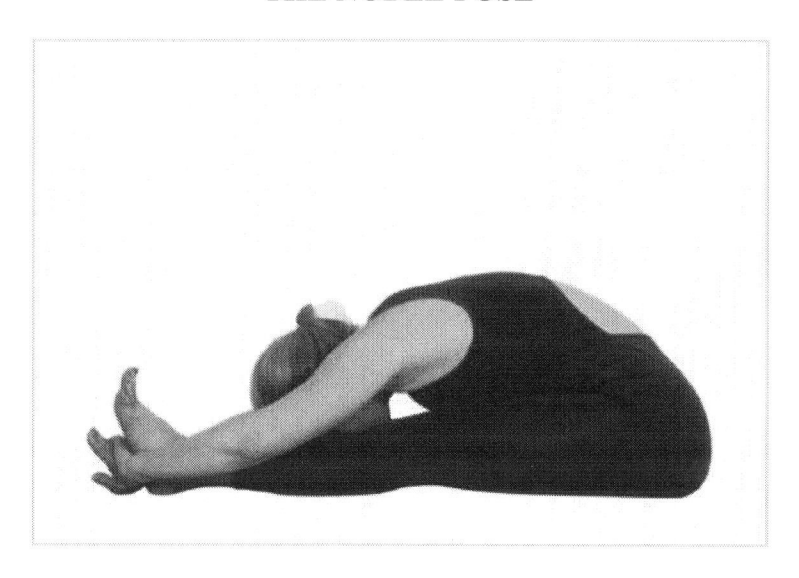

This pose stretches all the vertebrae of the spine and each muscle in the back. This type of stretching is highly beneficial. Blood flow to the abdominal region and tones the muscles increases as a result of the compression or contraction of the stomach. Sluggish digestion and constipation is also improved. The muscles in the calves and thighs get a good stretching, helping to relieve fatigue and soreness in the lower extremities.

THE SEATED FORWARD FOLD POSE

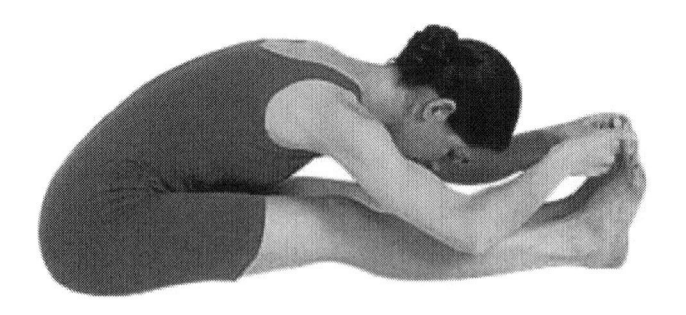

The pose has healing effect for high blood pressure, infertility and insomnia. It also assist a distracted mind relax. Also it helps in stretching the spinal column, shoulders, and hamstrings and also assists in stimulating the liver, kidneys, ovaries, and uterus. This pose reduces the symptoms of menopause and menstrual discomfort. This pose also calms the brain and relieves anxiety and soft depression.

THE BOUND ANGLE POSE

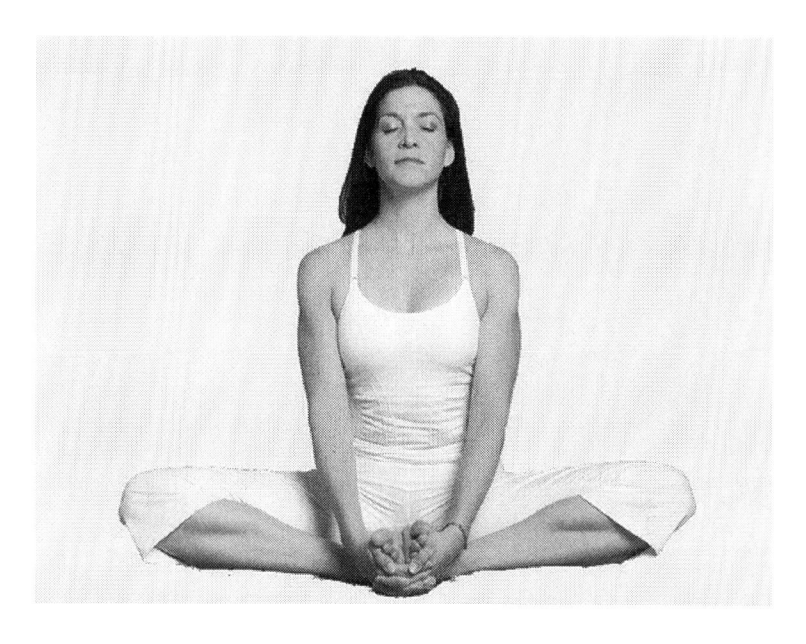

The pose is specifically recommended for pregnant women to practice until late into pregnancy as it ensures ease during childbirth. It is also has healing ability for high blood pressure, infertility, and asthma. It helps in stimulating the heart, abdominal organs, ovaries, prostate gland, bladder and kidneys. The pose improves general circulation and helps relieve soft depression, anxiety and weariness.

THE MOUNTAIN POSE

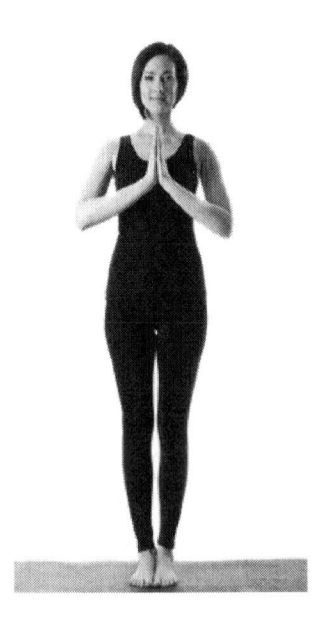

When this pose is performed properly and the mind is focused and free of distraction, the body is experienced as being rooted firmly to the earth and as steady and motionless as a mountain. Continual practice of the mountain pose along with other poses helps to re-train the body to stand correctly and reverse the negative effects of poor posture which causes discomforts, performing this pose allows one to observe one's posture closely and clearly recognize those problems which get ignored by day-to-day activities.

THE PLOW POSE

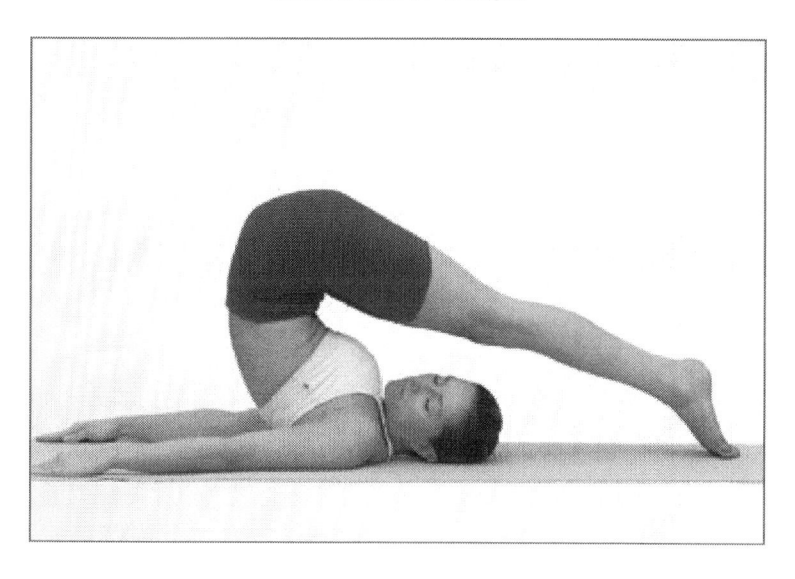

This pose stretches all the muscles and ligaments in the calves and thighs resulting in greater leg flexibility. It also relieves people of leg cramps. Since the abdominal area is contracted, blood compressed out of this area releases toxins and when the contraction is released the area is flooded with richly oxygenated blood. Repeating this pose will quickly restore suppleness to the spine as well as promote alertness.

THE TRIANGLE POSE

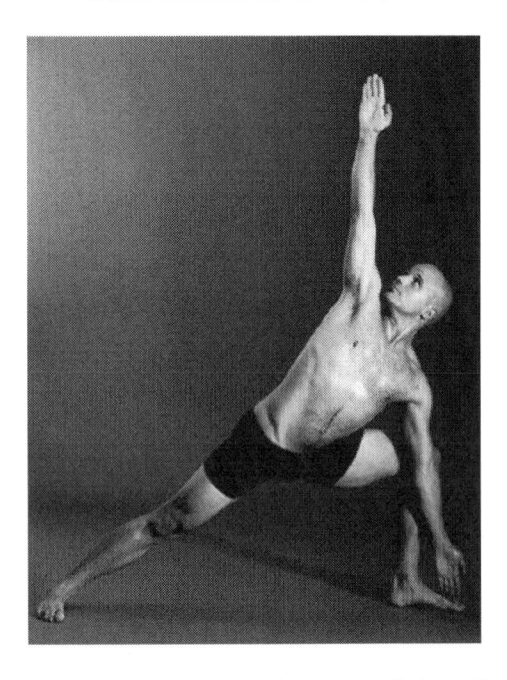

The forward bending and lifting when practicing the triangle pose stimulates blood flow and helps to stretch and relax the back, shoulders, legs and arms as well as increases the flow of blood to the head. The muscles of the thighs and calves as well as the hamstrings are stretched. The slight twist of the spine creates flexibility in the spinal discs and relieves lower back discomfort.

THE HEAD STAND POSE

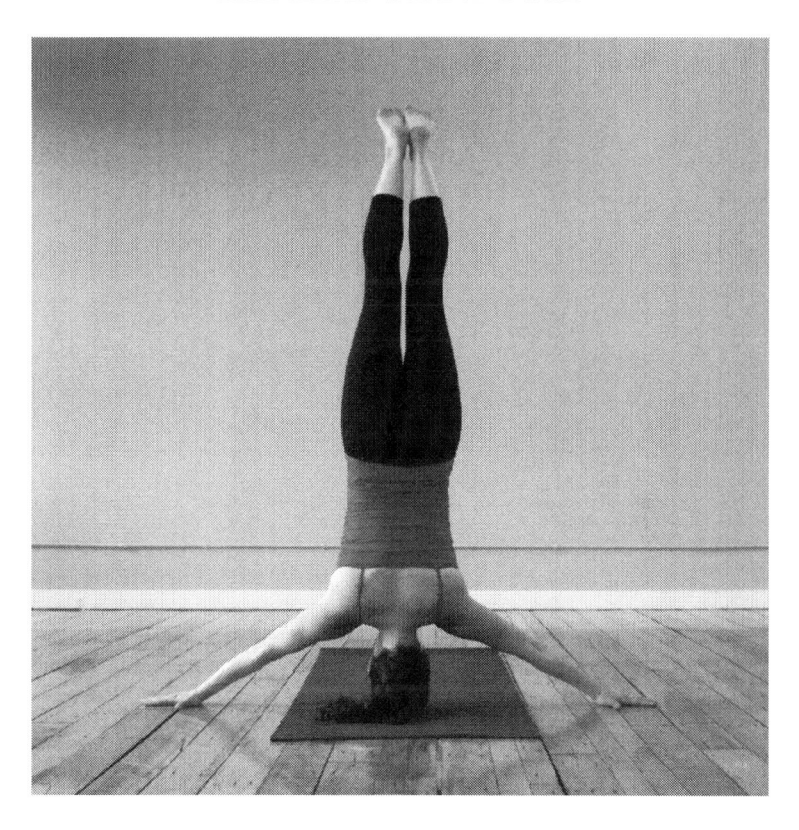

The Head-Stand Pose requires less flexibility of the legs yet it eases relaxation, concentration and in due course, meditation. It also helps to establish equilibrium throughout the body/mind. It will also help stretch the legs and pelvic area. The increased blood flow to the head and upper body helps to heal many disorders such as headaches, nasal congestion and sore throats.

THE SHOULDER STAND POSE

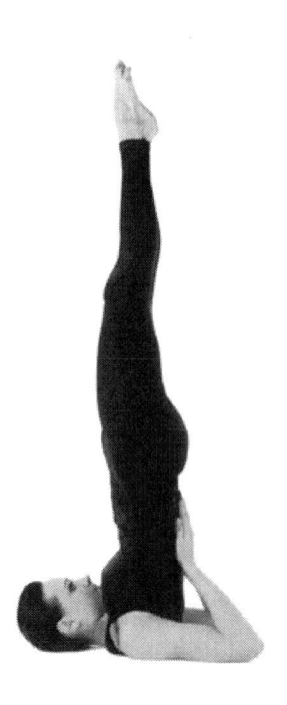

This pose provides great benefit to the abdominal organs helping to relieve gas and constipation and stimulate digestion. When performed in the morning the shoulder stand pose relieves fatigue caused by sleeping too much or too little and when practiced in the evening it promotes deep, restful sleep. The increased blood flow to the head and upper body helps to heal many disorders such as headaches, nasal congestion and sore throats.

THE LOWER BACK TWIST

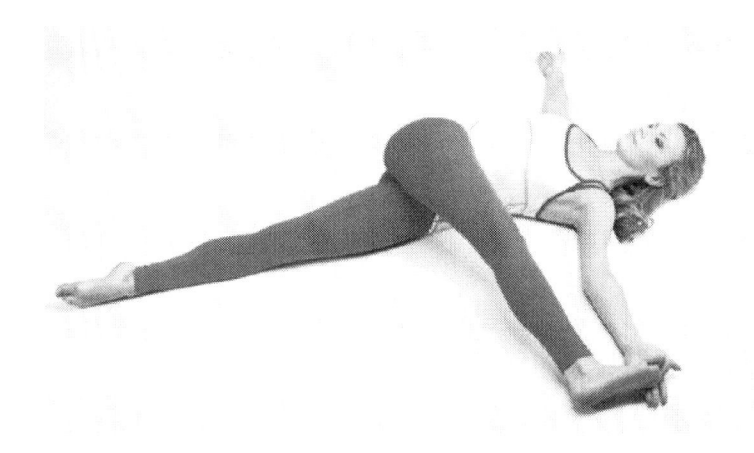

The lower back twist is one of the perfect poses to practice at the end of the Yoga session. It helps loosen the muscles and relaxing the spinal column. In the process of twisting the lower back the tension in this area is reduced. It also assists in lowering the blood pressure in patients with high blood pressure.

THE EASY BRIDGE POSE

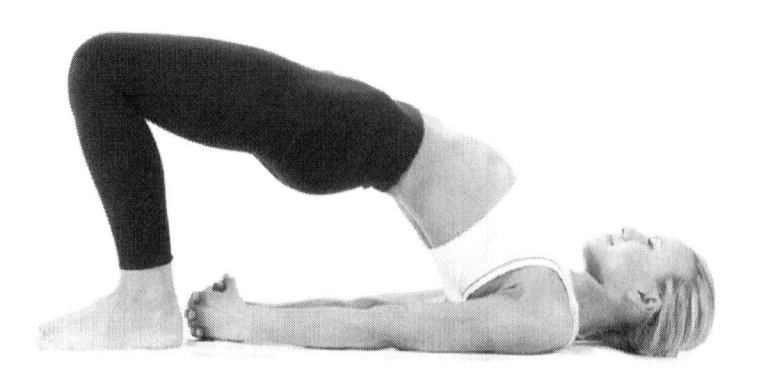

The easy bridge pose is very useful in easing stress, sciatica, headache and fatigue. It also plays a part in stimulating the abdominal organs, colon, lungs and thyroid glands, hence improving digestion. Constant practice often also revitalizes tired legs and has a slimming effect on both the thighs and buttocks.

THE CROCODILE POSE

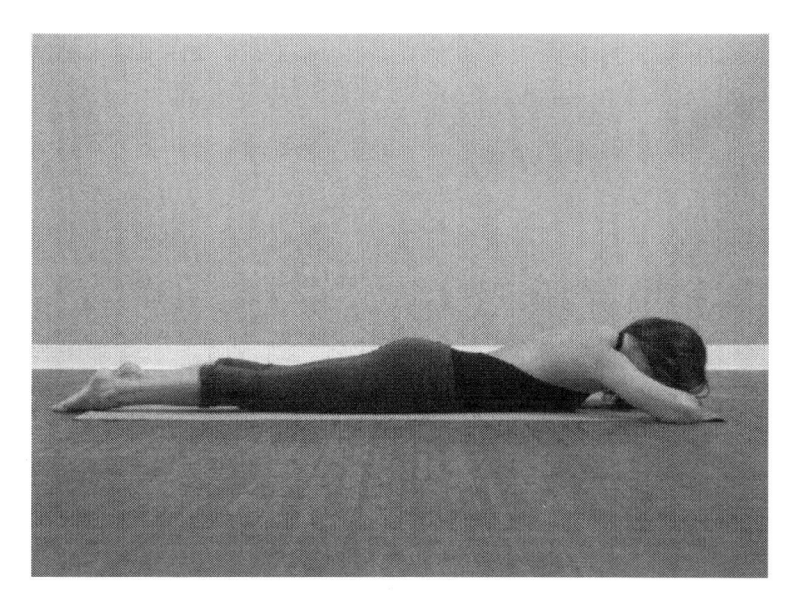

This pose has particularly been very effective for people suffering from slipped disc, sciatica and certain types of lower back pain. Being in this pose for extended periods of time pushes the vertebral column to resume its normal shape and also releases compression of the spinal nerves. It has also being helpful to people suffering from lungs ailment.

THE STANDING KNEE SIDE BALANCE POSE

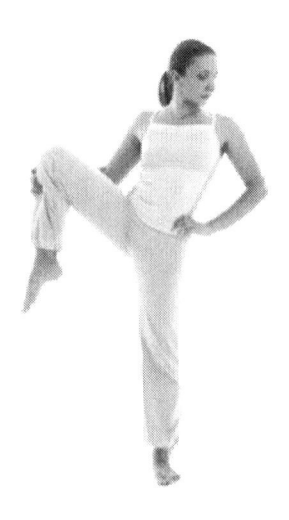

This particular pose is very helpful in developing both physical and mental stability. In the process of stretching the abdominal muscles and the intestines, the abdominal muscles and nerves are kept toned, hence, digestion is stimulated. Steady practice and improving the posture helps strengthen the arms and lower back

THE CHAIR POSE

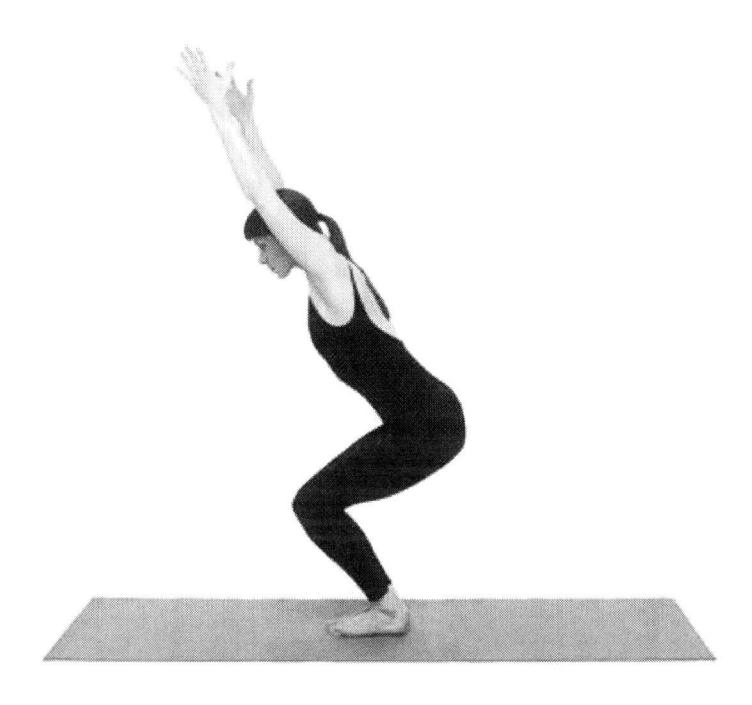

Regular practice of the Chair Pose keeps the abdominal organs and the back toned and the chest is developed by being fully expanded. It also helps in getting rid of inflexibility in the shoulders. The ankles become strong and the leg muscles develop evenly. The pose allows the diaphragm to be lifted up and this process gives a mild massage to the heart.

THE REVOLVED SIDE ANGLE STRETCH POSE

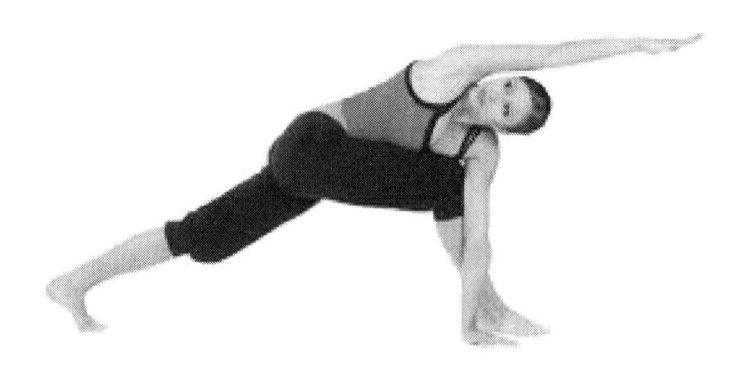

This pose has proved helpful when it comes to removing waste matter from the colon without strain. During this pose, the blood is distributed evenly across abdominal organs and the spinal column and they are thus revitalized. It is particularly helpful in improving digestion by contracting abdominal organs. It also helps in toning up ankles, knees and thighs

THE ONE LEG FORWARD BEND POSE I

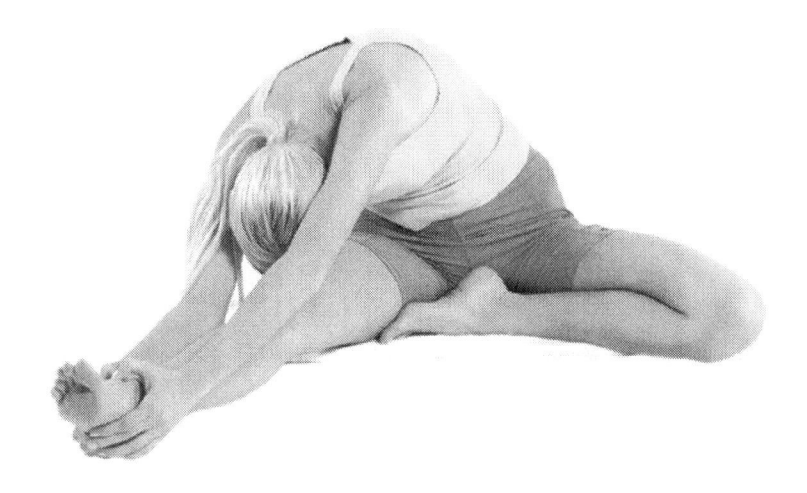

One of the major benefits of this pose is that it strengthens the legs. In addition, it opens up the hip and shoulders joints. It also helps in stretching the lower back; hence, it is helpful for treating sciatica. Contracting of the abdominal muscles during this pose helps to burn down the fat in this area.

THE ONE LEG FORWARD BEND POSE II

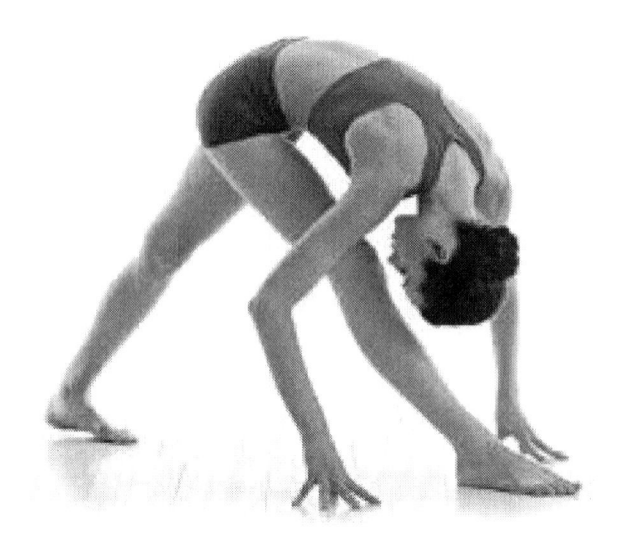

This pose is particularly recommended for removing excess weight in abdominal area and stimulating movement to the nerves and muscles of the spine. It plays a vital part in stretching hamstring muscles and gives room for flexibility in the hip joints. It assists in toning and massaging the entire abdominal and pelvic region.

THE WARRIOR POSE I

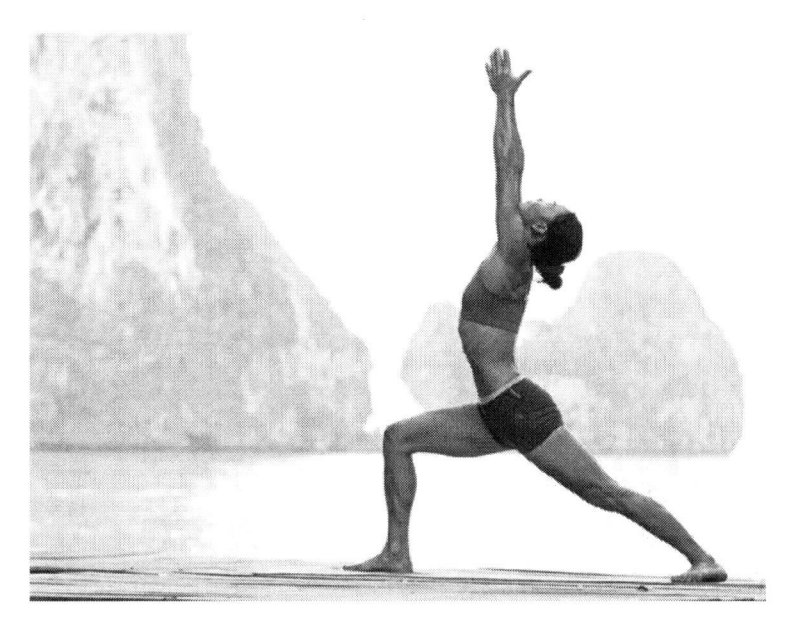

The warrior pose I help to develop good breathing in the chest and it also play a role in building stamina. Regular practice of the warrior pose strengthens the legs, ankles and knees. This pose has particularly helps in opening up and strengthening the shoulders, back and neck. It also assists in stretching the thighs.

THE WARRIOR POSE II

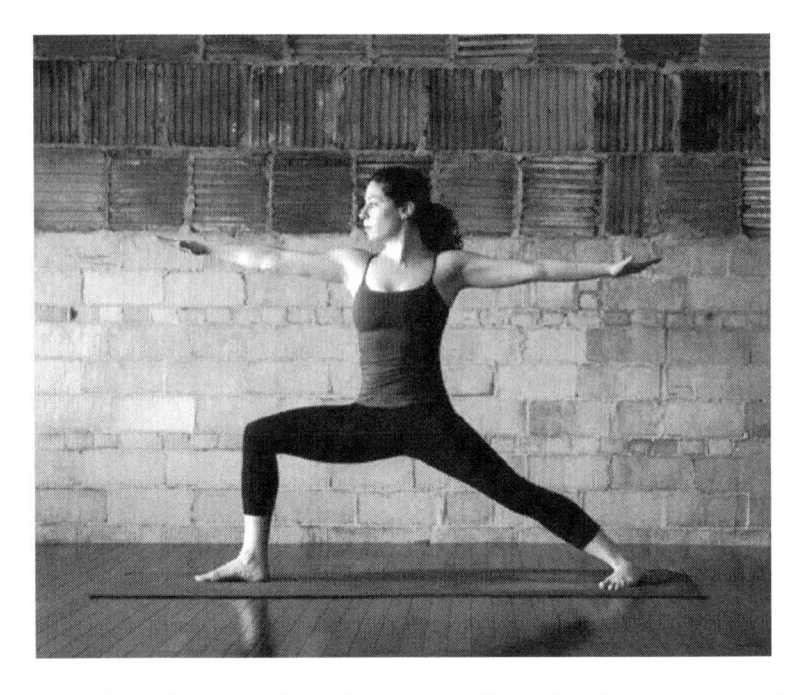

This pose has the same benefits as the first, but it also strengthens and shapes the legs, relieves leg cramps, brings flexibility to the legs and back, tones the abdomen, and strengthens the ankles and arms. It also assists in bringing elasticity to the legs and back muscles. It helps to develop good breathing in the chest too.

THE WARRIOR POSE III

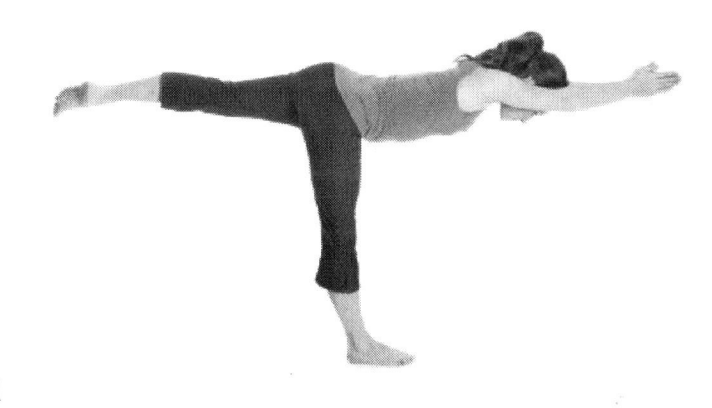

1

This warrior pose position develops the strength and shape of your legs and abdomen; it also gives you agility, poise, better concentration, and improved balance. Contracting and toning abdominal organs and making the leg muscles more shapely and sturdy are also made possible through regular practice. It is also helpful in getting rid of fat in abdominal area and hips.

THE LOTUS POSE

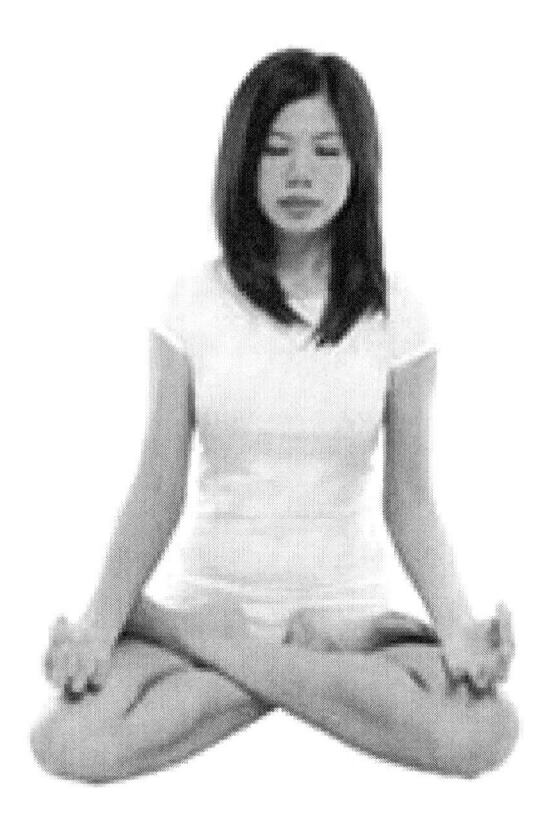

The lotus pose helps to aid relaxation, concentration and finally, meditation. The pose creates a natural balance throughout the body/mind. It is healthy, especially for those suffering from tired and aching muscles. It can be practiced directly after meals, for at least 5 minutes to enhance the digestive function. It helps in relieving stomach ailments such as hyperacidity and peptic ulcer

THE BOUND ANGLE POSE

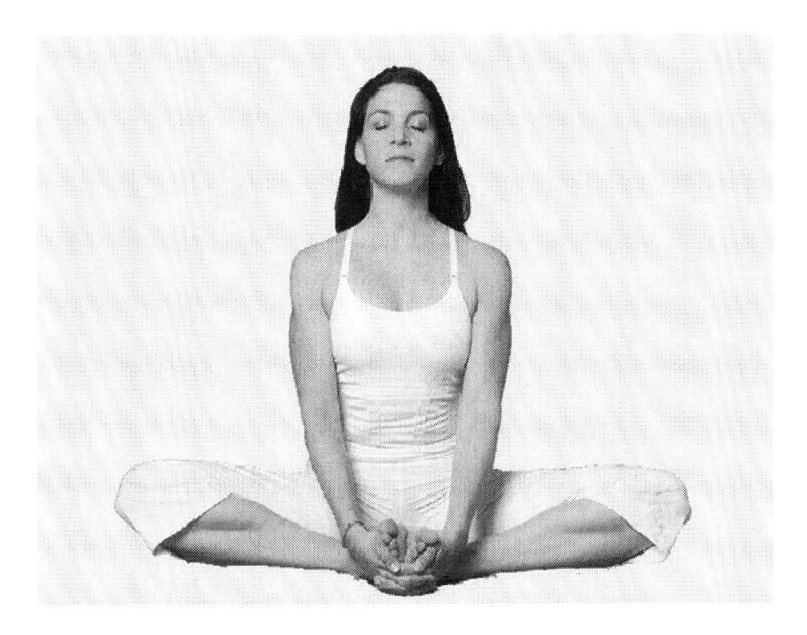

Bound Angle pose is an effective way of stimulating the heart, abdominal organs, ovaries, prostate gland, bladder and kidneys. Researched also proved that regular practise of this pose until late into pregnancy is said to help to make childbirth less difficult; hence, it is recommended for pregnant women. The pose improves general circulation and helps relieve mild depression, anxiety and fatigue.

THE FISH POSE

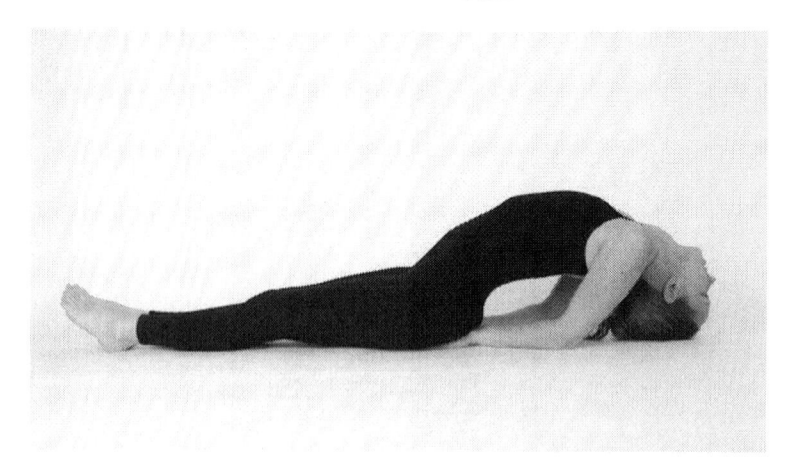

Practicing the fish pose causes a great expansion and stretching of the chest which aids in reducing upper respiratory congestion as-well-as benefits the heart. Furthermore, the sinus are drained and opened from the inversion of the head, stretching of the neck and pressure placed on the top of the head. It also helps in stimulating the thyroid and parathyroid glands.

THE BUTTERFLY POSE

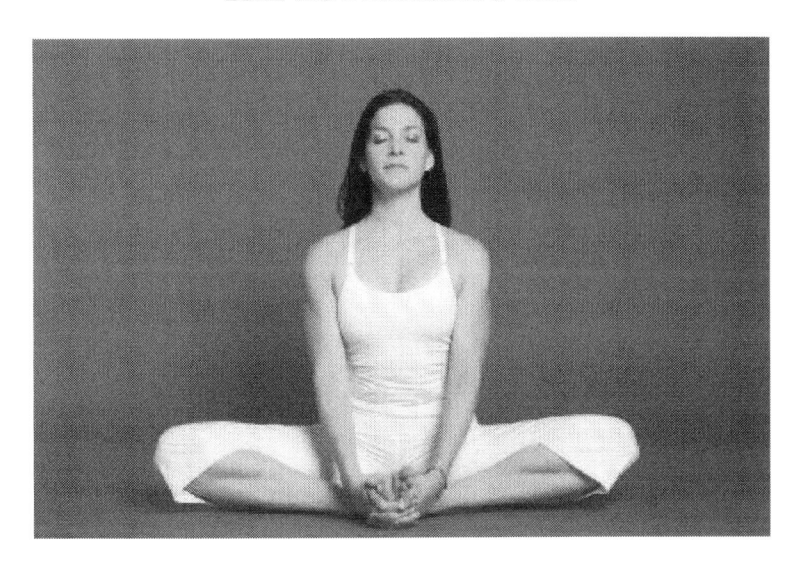

The Butterfly pose helps improves the flexibility in the groin and reduces the stiffness around the hips region. It has proved to be helpful in relieving the inner thigh muscles tension and also helps removes tiredness from long hours of walking or standing. It is also a recommended pose for preparing the legs for other meditative postures.

THE TWISTED FORWARD STRETCH POSE

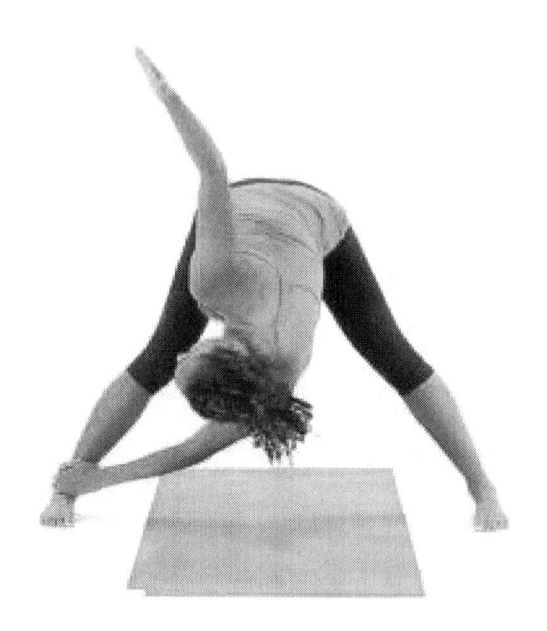

It helps in stretching the hamstring muscles and also gives room for flexibility of the hip joints. Regular practice results in toning of the abdominal muscles. The arms and spine muscles are also strengthened through constant practice of this pose. This pose causes a gentle twist to occur at the lower back which helps in strengthening lower back muscles.

THE LOCUST POSE

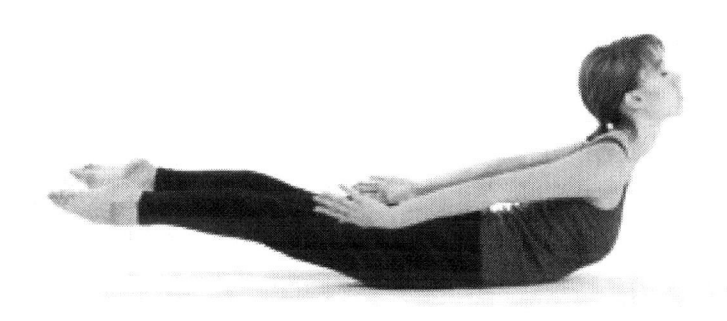

The Locust pose tones and balances the functioning of the liver, stomach, bowels, and other abdominal organs. If done properly it helps in tightening the muscles of the buttocks. Regular practice helps in strengthening the lower back; hence, recommended for people suffering from sciatica. It is effective for correcting poor posture and also helps relieve stress.

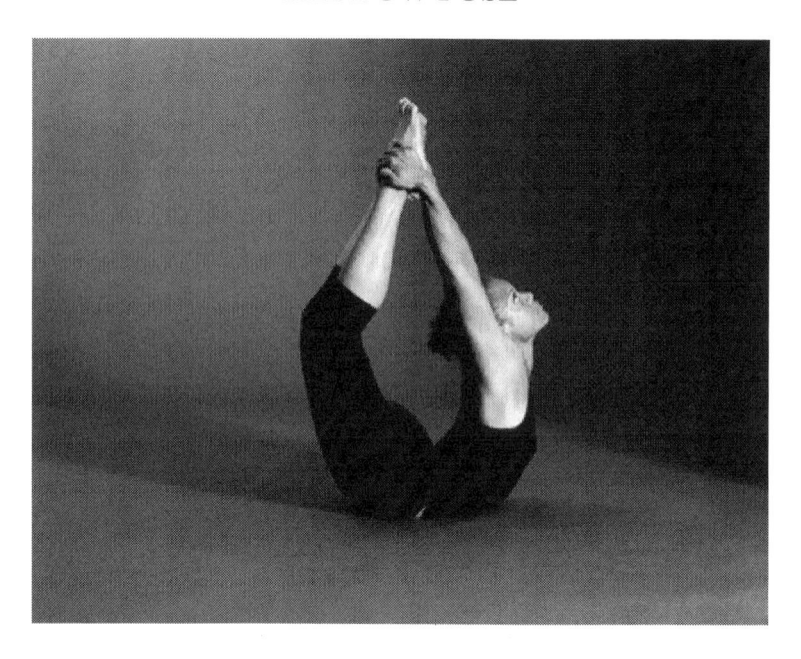

THE BOW POSE

The Bow Pose has proved to be a very effective and the best yoga pose to burn belly fat. It influences toning and stretching the entire front of the body, ankles, abdomen, thighs, chest and throat, spine. If correctly done it helps improve the functioning of the digestive organs. It strengthens leg muscles, especially thighs too.

THE COBRA POSE

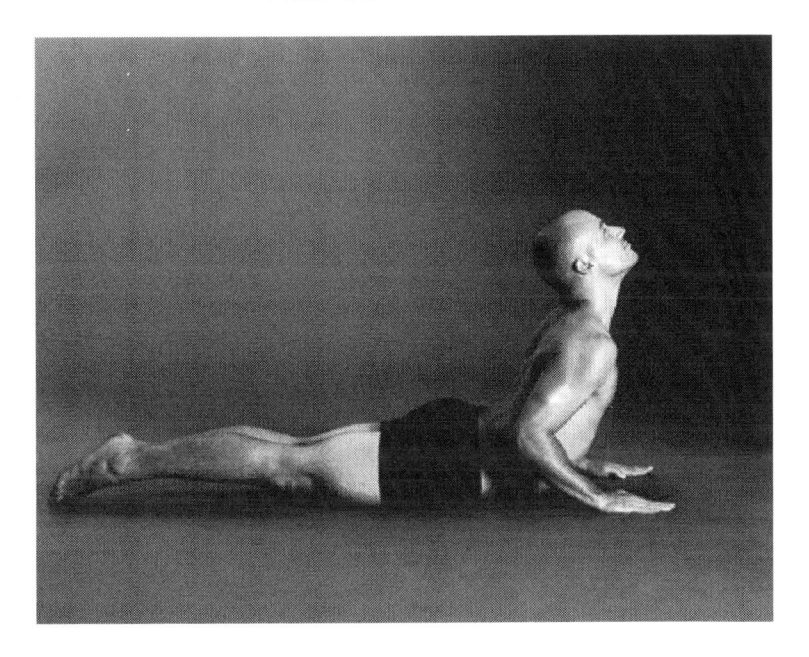

It helps reduce the effects of backache and also allows the spine maintains its flexibility. It eases constipation and is beneficial for all abdominal organs, especially the liver and kidneys. The spine, chest, abdomen, shoulders are strengthened through consistent practice. It also helps to keep the buttocks firm and stiffened. It is a recommended pose for heart and lungs opening.

THE CHILD POSE

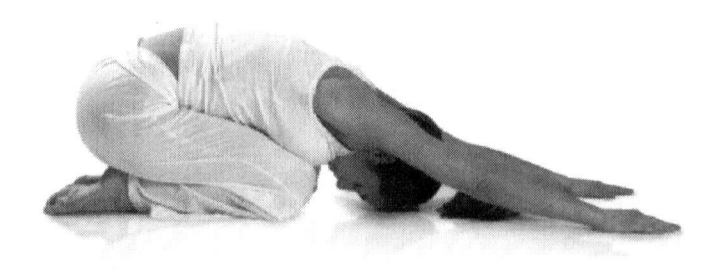

The child pose is often practiced after Sun Salutations and in between sequences. Its soothing effect helps you relax, calm down, relieve stress and fatigue and on the long run helps stretch the hips, thighs and ankles. It restores balance in the body and tends to release tension in the back, shoulders, and chest.

THE CAT POSE

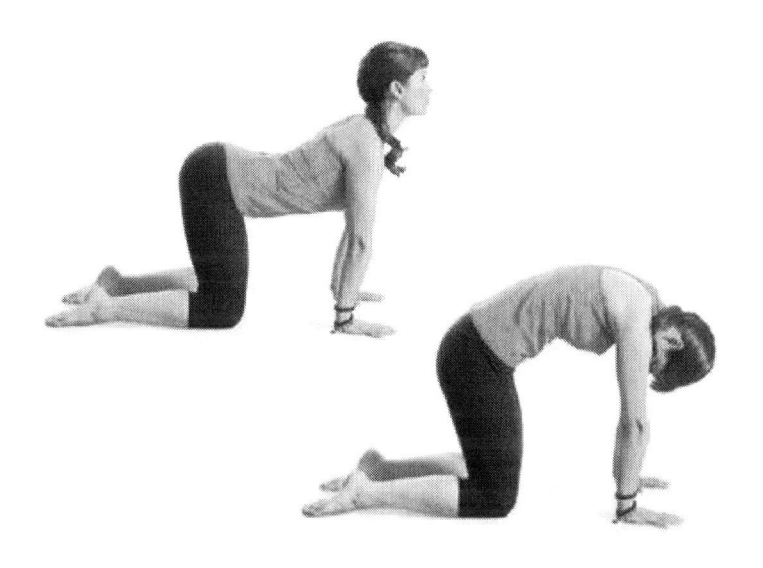

The pressure applied on the lower abdomen when doing the pose helps to tone the digestive system muscles. The pose has some massaging effect on the spine and abdomen and it also develops the wrists and arms. The cat pose aids making the neck, shoulders and spine maintains its flexibility.

THE DOWNWARD FACING DOG POSE

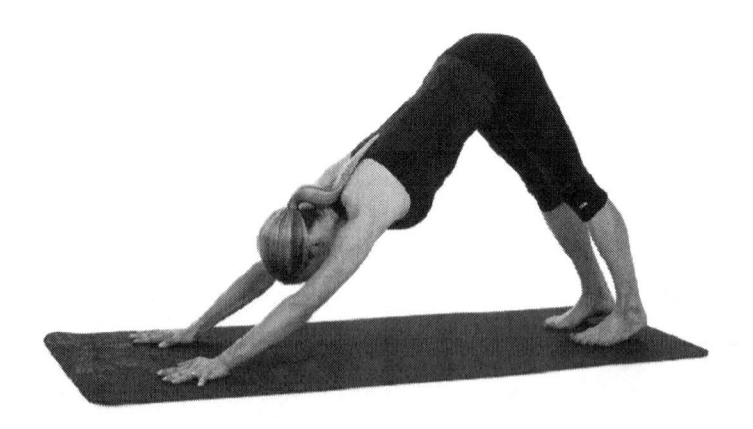

The downward facing dog pose has been beneficial in helping the brain relax and relieving tension. It has also proven to energize the body. The arms, shoulders, hamstrings and calf are also stretched in the process. It has a slimming effect on arms and legs. It aids in improving digestion, relieving headache, insomnia, back pain and fatigue.

THE RAISED LEG DOWNWARD FACING DOG POSE

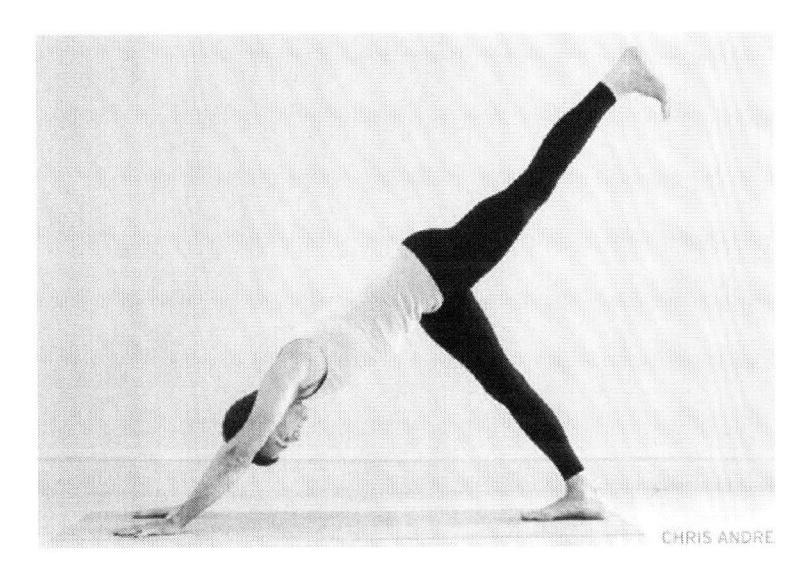

The Raised Leg downward facing dog pose has similar benefits with the downward facing dog pose like in helping the brain relax and relieving tension. It also helps energize the body. The arms, shoulders, hamstrings and calf are also stretched in the process. It has a slimming effect on arms and legs. Its benefits also include strengthening the nerves and muscles in the limbs and back.

THE TIPTOE POSE

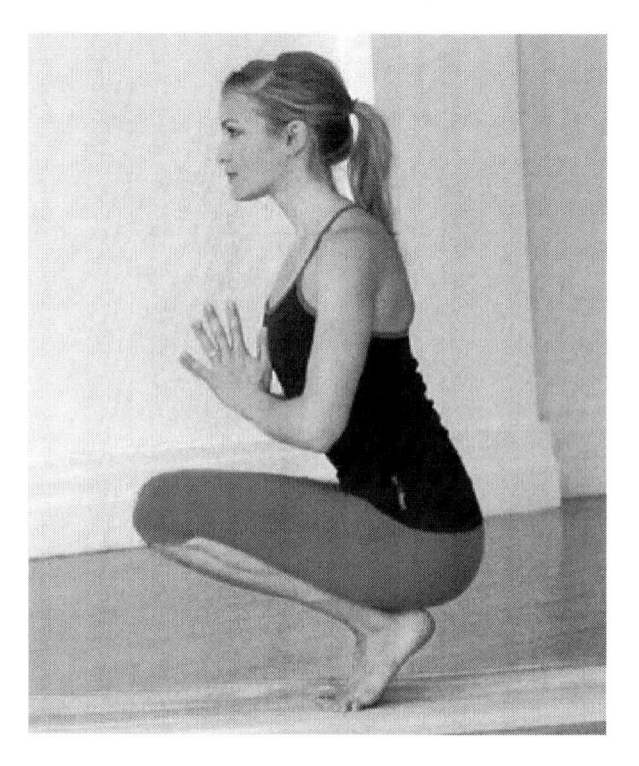

Aside the fact that the tip toe pose improves both mental and physical balance and also increases concentration, this pose is improves strength and flexibility in the toes, abdominal muscles, ankles, lower back and thighs. It also helps develop stronger joints, which helps to improve arthritis and knee pain.

THE CHEST EXPAND POSE

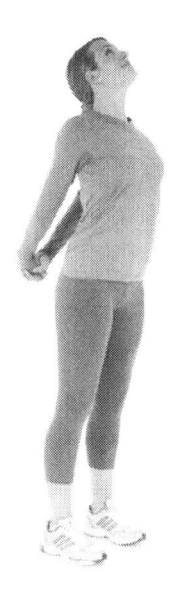

In addition to the chest expand pose being able to strengthen the hand, arm, shoulder and back it helps to stretch the arms and spine and helps to counteract a rounded back. The pose is beneficial in the sense that it helps to deepen the breath. Consistent practice makes it useful in toning abdominal muscles.

THE SIDE PLANK POSE

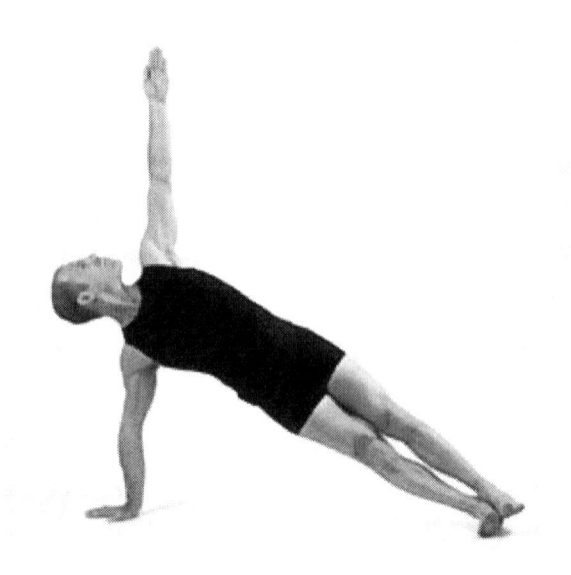

The benefits of the side plank pose include strengthening your shoulders, upper back, and abdominals. It also promotes core and scapular stability, which is helpful if you working on inversions or arm balance. It stretches and strengthens the wrists and legs. It is also a good pose for improving balance and coordination.

THE DOLPHIN POSE

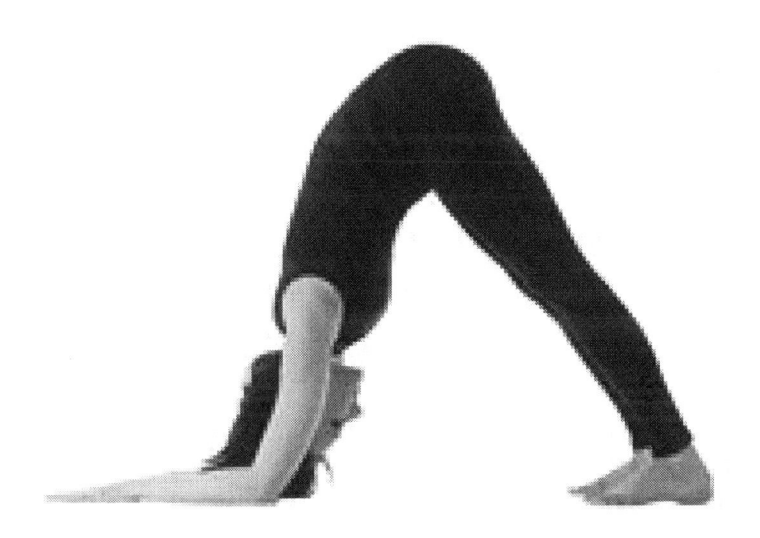

The dolphin pose helps build strength in the upper body in preparations for other poses like the headstand and forearm stand pose. It can also help calm the mind, relieve stress and to relieve back pain and to cure mild depression. It is a good pose for regulating digestion and toning of core muscles. It is helpful in stretching the hamstrings, calves and arches.

THE SURRENDER POSE

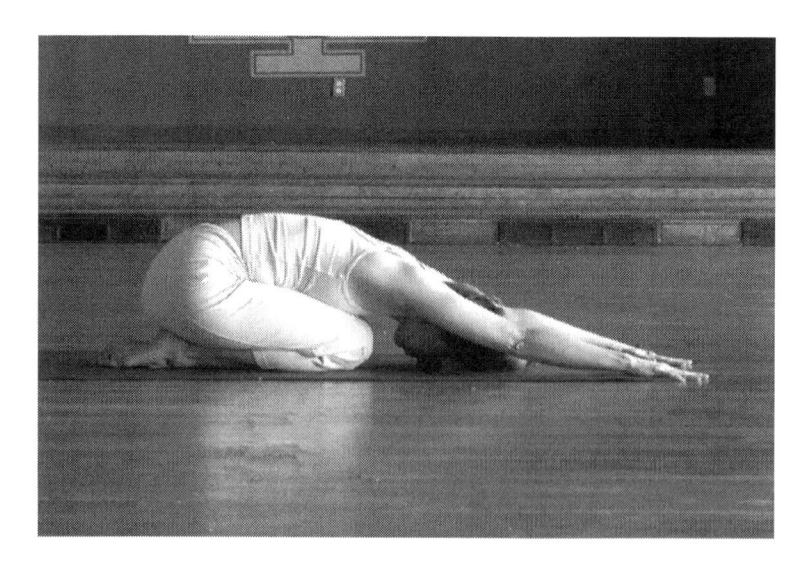

The surrender pose is very useful for relaxing the body and helpful when it comes to relieving tension from the lower back and arms. In addition, it strengthens the abdominal muscles, digestive system and spine muscles. If done regularly and properly, it applies pressure on the abdominal organs and this helps stimulate digestion.

THE EXTENDED SIDE ANGLE STRETCH POSE

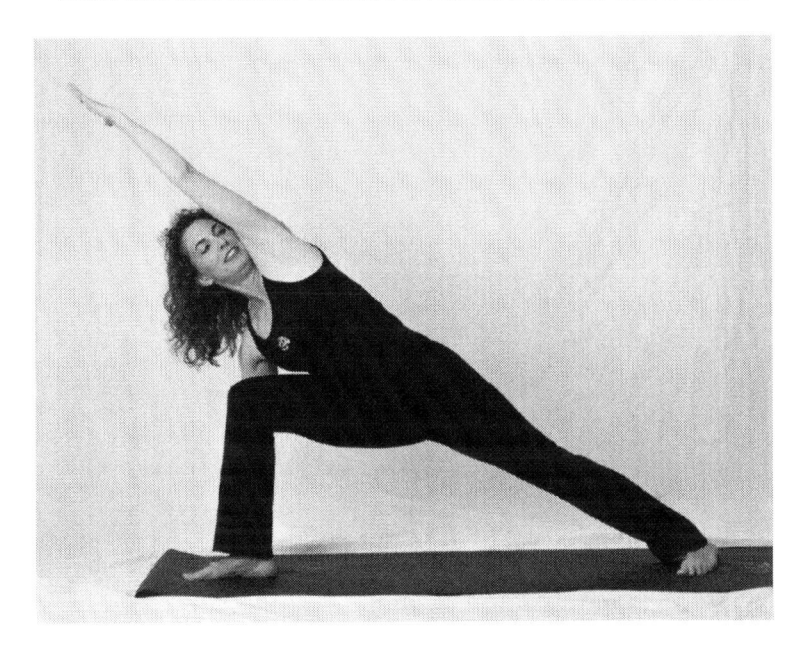

This pose has particularly been beneficial because it helps the back to turn more and create a deeper stretch along the spine. It also helps strengthen the thighs, knees, hips and ankles. It massages and stimulates the abdominal organs. The groin, back, spine, waist, ankles, lungs (intercostals) and shoulders are also stretched.

THE WIDE LEG FORWARD BEND POSE

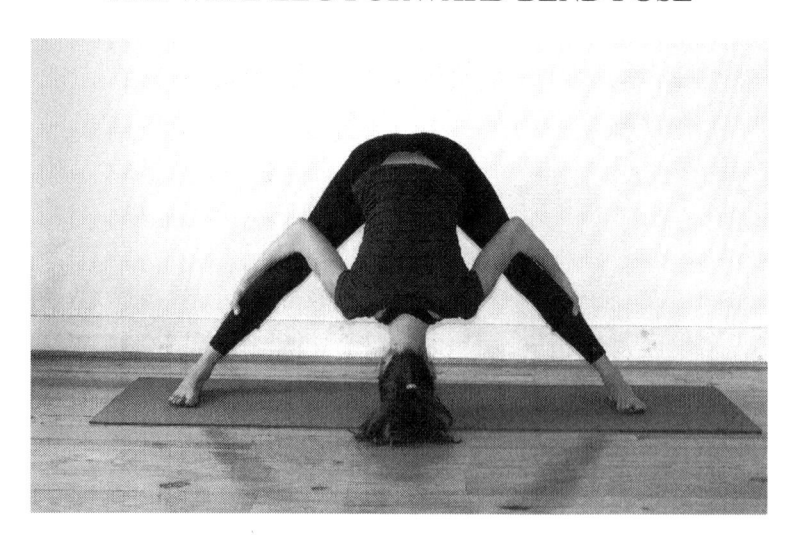

The wide leg forward pose has several benefits which include: Stretching the groins, hamstrings and hips. It also decompresses the spine and relives fatigue, mild depression and anxiety. It aids in strengthening and slimming the arms and upper back. It is very useful in calming the mind.

THE HALF MOON POSE

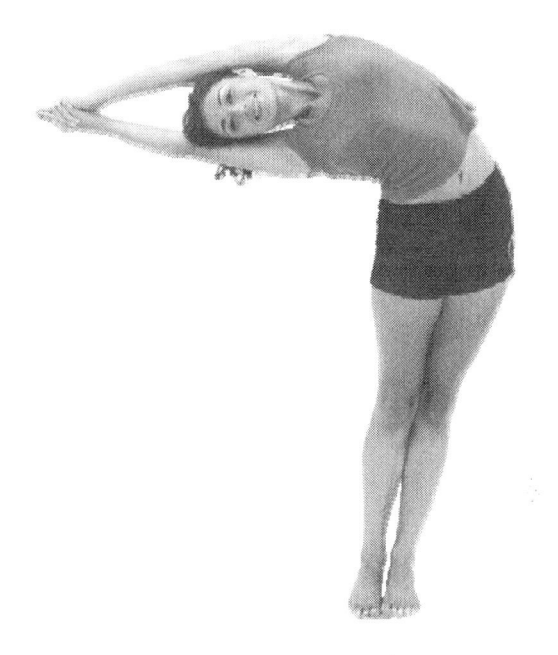

The half-moon pose improves balance, focus, concentration and confidence. It opens the hips and helps strengthen the ankles, knees and the lower body. It also helps to reduce the fat around the hips. It stretches the hamstrings, calfs and thighs muscles. Consistent practice helps in toning the buttock.

THE RABBIT POSE

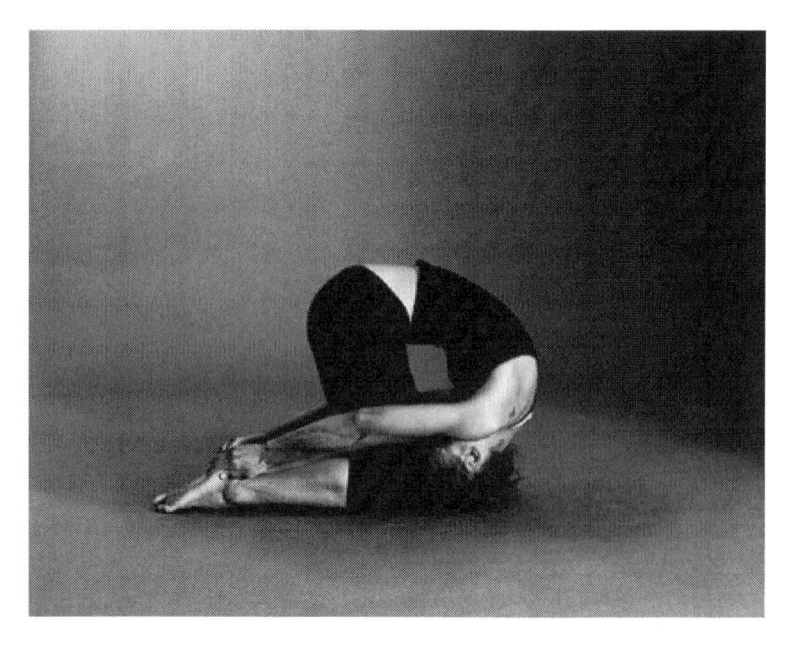

This pose produces the same effect as the camel pose; as a result, it stretches the spine to permit the nervous system to receive proper nutrition. It also helps to keep the mobility and elasticity of the spine and back muscles in check. It relieves digestion and helps sinus problems, and chronic tonsillitis. It improves the flexibility of the scapula.

THE HEAD TO KNEE POSE WITH STRETCHING POSE

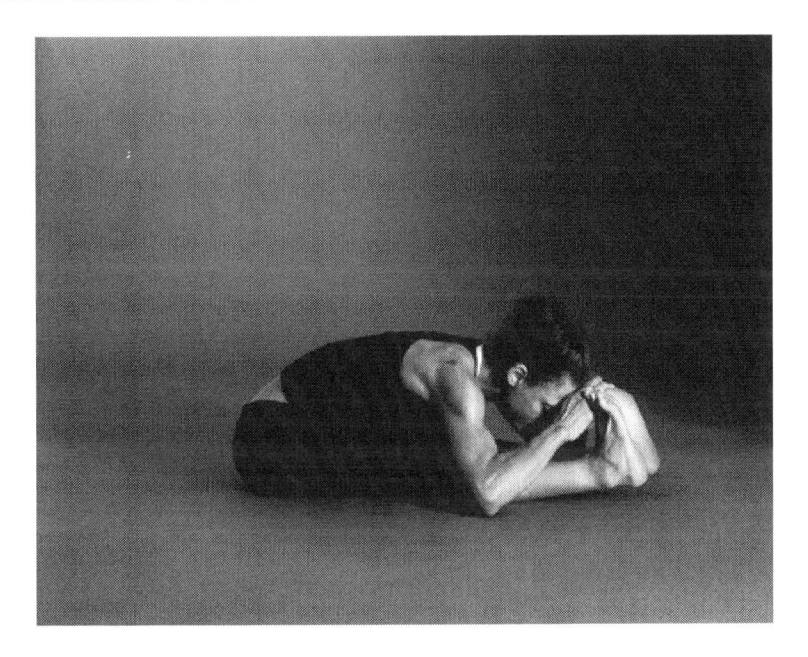

This pose increases the flexibility of the trapezius as well as the sciatic nerves, tendons, hip joints, and the last five major vertebrae of the spine. It also helps to keep the blood sugar levels in check and plays a role in enhancing the proper function of the kidneys. It improves digestion; hence, helps relieve chronic diarrhea.

THE STANDING BOW PULLING POSE

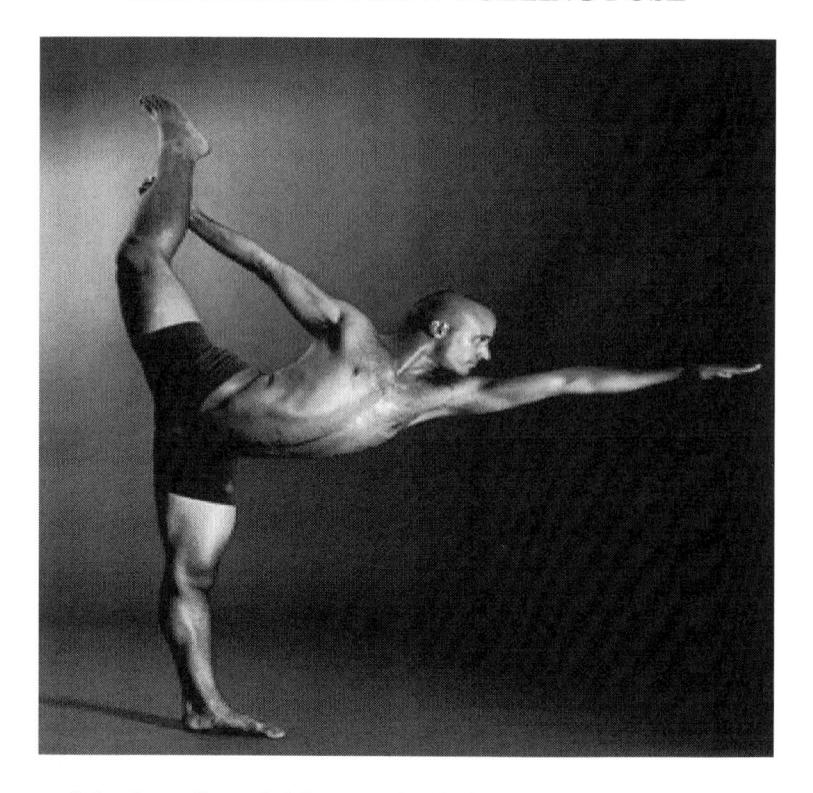

Some of the benefits of this pose includes: improving flexibility and strength of the spine, legs, hips and shoulders. It tightens abdominal and thigh muscles, it also tightens the arms, hips and buttocks. The pose helps to develop mental determination and develop balance. It also improves posture, while increasing elasticity of the rib cage and the lungs.

THE HALF TORTOISE POSE

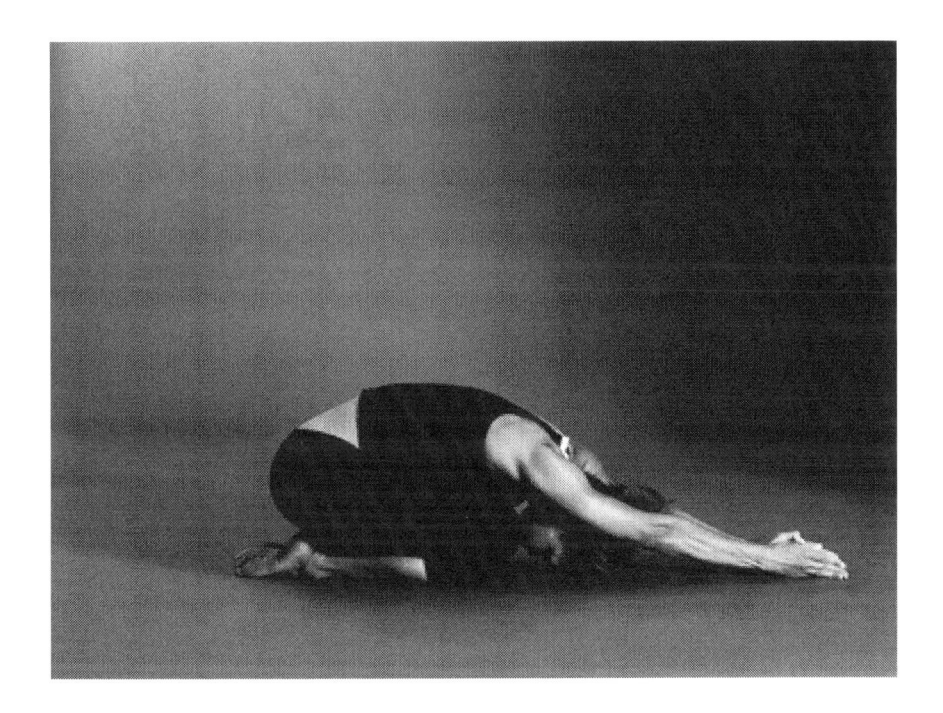

The Half tortoise pose helps provide maximum relaxation and aids indigestion and stretches the lower part of the lungs, increasing blood circulation to the brain. It also makes the abdomen and thighs firm. The pose helps to increase the flexibility of hip joints, scapula, deltoids, triceps, and latisimus dorsi muscles.

THE BALANCING STICK POSE

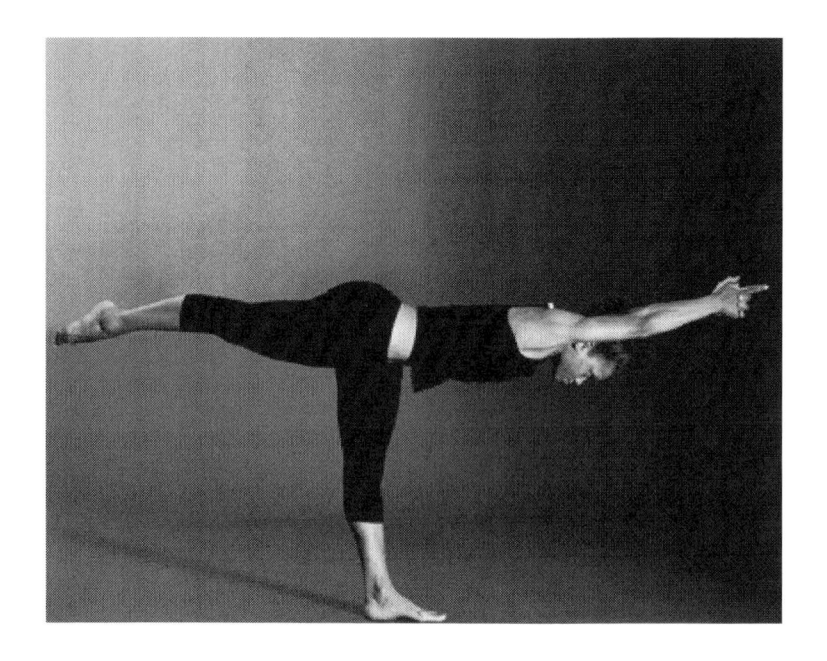

The pose perfects control and balance. It helps firm the hips, buttocks, and upper thighs, as well as providing many of the same benefits for the legs as in Standing Head to Knee. Increases circulation and strengthens the cardiovascular system, this is an excellent exercise for poor posture. Improves flexibility, strength, and muscle tone of shoulders, upper arms, spine, and hip joints.

2 WEEK SCHEDULE TO INCREASE RELAXATION

Sleep deprivation and stress can be a sadistic cycle. The fact that we don't relax after having a hectic day makes us stressed the next day. That's where yoga comes into play. By relaxing, and relieving tension in the body, the soothing practice can be an effective relaxation remedy. The following relaxation poses if practiced every day of the week can be particularly helpful for combating restlessness and insomnia, especially when practiced in the evening or in bed before hitting the hay. Here is a weekly schedule of yoga poses or programs that can be done every day of the week to get rid of stress and help relax the mind. Each pose or program can be practiced for at least 15mins each day.

Sunday – Spine twisting pose

Monday – Easy Forward Bend.

Tuesday – Standing Forward Bend

Wednesday – Child Pose

Thursday – Plow Pose

Friday – Corpse Pose

Saturday – Left Nostril breathing

3 WEEK SCHEDULE TO INCREASE FLEXIBILITY

Flexibility is a vital part of staying in good health and maintaining it. The stretching done during yoga exercises is a great way to improve your flexibility. Doing yoga regularly is a sure way to become more flexible. If that's your aim, here are some poses that target major muscles groups that tend to get tight from sitting for long periods or even from other types of exercise, like running. Staying in the poses for several minutes is the way to get a good stretch. Don't expect overnight changes, however. For best results, do your stretches daily. The following poses are intended to give you some options to fit your current level of flexibility.

Mountain Pose – It looks simple but it is a basic outline for all other postures. It is a good start-up pose.

Standing Forward Bend and the Triangle Pose are some essential poses for improving flexibility in the hamstring. Also Downward facing dog pose also helps in preparing you for the real flexibility yoga practice.

You can follow this flexibility schedule every day. Each pose can be practiced for at least 15 minutes each day

Sunday-Chair pose

Monday- Tree pose

Tuesday- Bridge pose

Wednesday-locust pose

Thursday- Warrior II pose and the

Friday- Plank pose

Saturday- Mountain pose

The above schedule scan help make you flexible if practiced consistently for every day of the week.

4 WEEK SCHEDULE TO IMPROVE BREATHING

Yoga usually involves paying attention to your breath, which can help you relax. It may also call for specific breathing techniques. But yoga typically isn't aerobic, like running or cycling, unless it's an intense type of yoga or you're doing it in a heated room. Yoga involves relaxing in different postures while keeping focus on the breath. As a result, every yoga posture has a particular effect on the heart; and therefore affecting the heart as well.

Here are some poses that can be practiced every day of the week to improve breathing and keep the heart running effectively.

These poses begin with mild ones, gradually increasing to more demanding ones that require greater stamina and strength. The body gets relaxed and rejuvenated with the concluding postures.

Mountain Pose, Tree Pose, Triangle Pose, Warrior Pose, Chair Pose, Cat Pose, and Downward facing dog Pose are examples of poses that helps improve breathing. For a weekly schedule for breathing you can try these poses out for at least 15 minutes every day.

Sunday-Cobra Pose
Monday-Bow Pose
Tuesday-Bridge Pose
Wednesday-Two leg forward bend
Thursday-Plank Pose
Friday-Dolphin Pose
Saturday-Corpse Pose

5 WEEK SCHEDULE TO INCREASE MENTAL FOCUS

As humans, there are lots of distractions and this makes it harder for us all to focus and be productive. A daily yoga practice does not only help you chill out, but also helps the mind to focus. It also has the capacity to alter the way you live and approach your life. Incorporate the following yoga poses in your everyday practice to build your concentration and focus.

There are some poses to counteract all of the blustery-ness and allow for maximum concentration. If you ever feel distracted and not focused, try each of these poses for 10-15 minutes every day of the week, go back to your task, and get the better of the world.

Sunday-Eagle Pose (this pose will not only be beneficial to increase your metal focus but it will also help release the tension from the shoulders and hips)

Monday-Mountain Pose

Tuesday-Standing forward Bend

Wednesday-Downward facing dog (is an important pose that aids to calm and focus a distracted mind. Focus on deep, full-body breaths and releasing and tension in the legs or back)

Thursday-Warrior I

Friday-Warrior III

Saturday-Corpse Pose

Printed in Great Britain
by Amazon